SELF-LOVE
THE POWER WITHIN
EVERY WOMAN

A Practical Self-Help Guide on Valuing Your Significance as a Woman of Power

Sensei Paul David

Copyright Page

Self-Love-The Power Within Every Woman, by Sensei
Paul David,
Copyright © 2021.

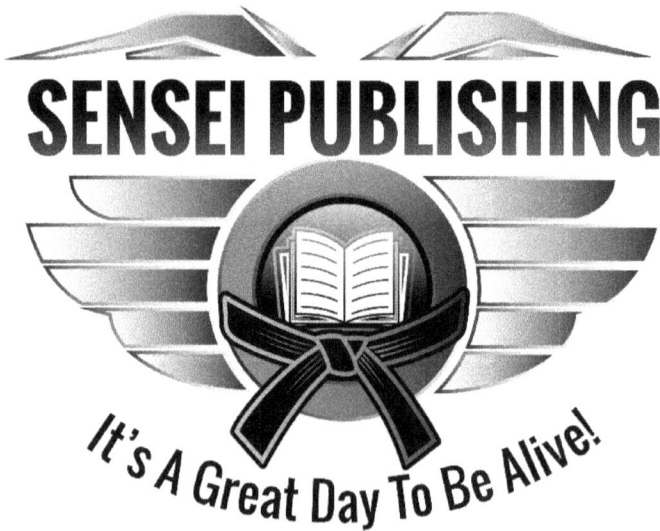

SENSEI PUBLISHING

It's A Great Day To Be Alive!

www.senseipublishing.com

@senseipublishing
#senseipublishing

Get/Share Our FREE All-Ages Mental Health Books Now!

FREE Kids Books

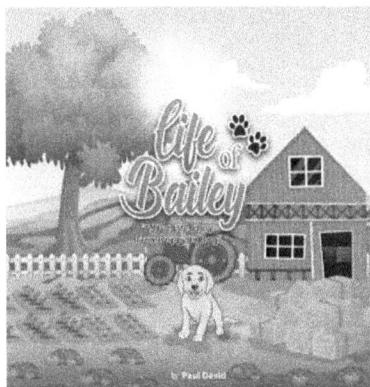

lifeofbailey.senseipublishing.com

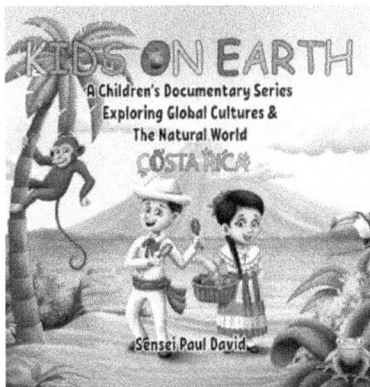

kidsonearth.senseipublishing.com

FREE Self-Development Book for Every Family

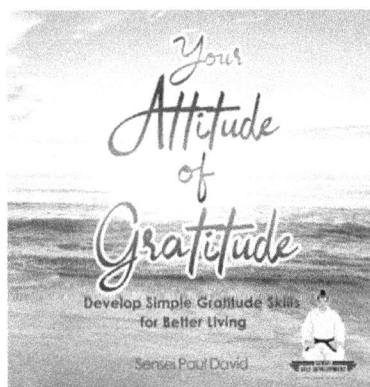

senseiselfdevelopment.senseipublishing.com

Click Below or Search Amazon for Another Book In Each Series Or Visit:

www.amazon.com/author/senseipauldavid

KIDS ON EARTH

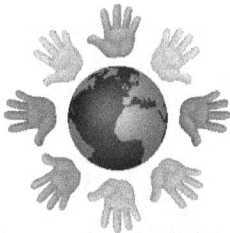

kidsonearth.senseipublishing.com

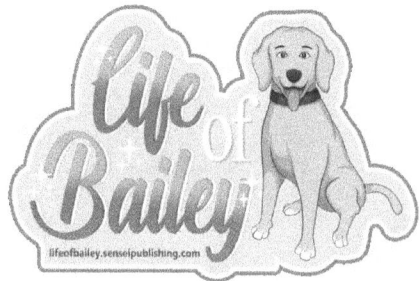

lifeofbailey.senseipublishing.com

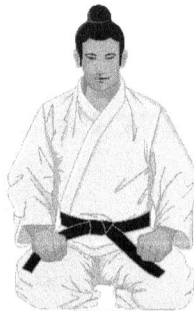

SENSEI SELF DEVELOPMENT
BOOKS SERIES
senseiselfdevelopment.senseipublishing.com

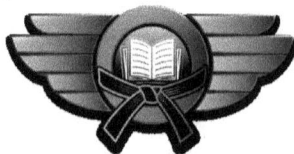

Join Our Publishing Journey!

If you would like to receive FUTURE FREE BOOKS, and get to know us better, please click www.senseipublishing.com and join our newsletter by entering your email address in the pop-up box.

Follow Our Blog: senseipauldavid.ca

Follow/Like/Subscribe: Facebook, Instagram, YouTube: @senseipublishing

Scan the QR Code with your phone or tablet

to follow us on social media: Like / Subscribe / Follow

FOREWORD

You would probably think that it is unusual to read a book about women's self-development that is written by a man. Given that I am not a woman myself, I don't claim to be an expert in this field.

Nevertheless, I do have a deep respect for women and so, this book represents my genuine attempt at providing specific emotional value to women, inspired by my appreciation for people as a whole.

For the daughters, mothers, and sisters in the world, this book is indeed written for you.

I hope you will find assurance in yourself of the value you are looking for and a more effective exposition of love that you can offer to others, especially to your loved ones.

Thank You from The Author: Sensei Paul David

Before we dive in, I would like to thank you for picking up this book from among the many other similar books out there. Thank you for choosing to invest in my book. That means everything to me.

Now that you are here, I ask you to stick with me as we take your self-discovery journey together. I promise to make our time together valuable and worthwhile.

In the pages ahead, you will find some areas of information and practices more helpful than others - and that is great! I encourage you to apply what works best for you. You will benefit from the knowledge that you gain and the ensuing exciting transformation of character. Enjoy!

Contents

Introduction

"Love yourself first and everything falls into line."

Think of how much the world of today demands more of you—your time, attention, efforts, ideas, and almost everything about you. And you start *giving* it all, little by little.

You start pouring everything of yourself into whatever is demanded of you. It may be grilling your time for work, loving the person on the other end of your relationship that is obviously toxic or losing your rest over serving other people.

The present time seems to cram you out and leave you exhausted in bed at night, only to find yourself flustered by the alarm clock in the morning.

As a woman, you have to be strong because this world does not allow any weak creature to survive. And so, you are getting to the point of losing everything, including yourself.

And yes, this is not healthy. You know it, yet you have still been losing out on time for yourself. You think you don't deserve any shut-eye for some reason.

Or maybe your triggering inferiority complex brought you here to find this book.

You feel like you are less than others existing in this world, and even your own breath does not matter in any way to you.

Self-love is a word so impossible for you to grasp. It is a word so far from your level of perception. So, you are apathetic towards yourself, which then also extends to others around you.

Maybe that's precisely why you picked up this book. And that is the best decision you have made for yourself so far.

Either of the reasons I have laid out or whatever it is that brought you here, dear woman, I am sure you want to love yourself more in a way you've never known possible.

But I must give you a heads-up. Self-love would only be out of your reach if, by any means, you neglect it, saying you do not need it or there is no time for that.

It seems impossible for those who don't believe in such love. Therefore, before diving into this profound journey of learning more about how to love yourself, you must examine yourself first.

Are you here to condemn yourself through self-pity?

Or are you here to finally surrender all the doubts, hatred, and apathy towards, and about yourself, and rewrite your story into something marvellous and colourful?

Go on, spoil yourself with a good rest on the couch or on your bed and keep reading.

I hope this book will not only fill the enormous void in your heart about loving yourself but will honestly change the way you think about yourself.

Knowing and loving who you are will change the way you view the world around you.

And guess what—another heads-up—even desiring to finish this book will definitely mean that you are starting to love yourself, hoping for a change of heart and mind.

While we're at it, you can enjoy the benefits of this book by searching your identity first. Perhaps, you should ask yourself: What changes do I want to see, the moment I take this journey through this book?

With that, you are ready to dive deep into the wonders of self-love, specially written for you.

What does self-love mean?

I guess we would actually think that it's as easy to love oneself as the two connected words suggest. And I won't argue with that.

Nevertheless, we would want to expand the words further to totally grasp what it means to love oneself, despite everything that keeps one from doing it.

Self-love is simply knowing who you are; accepting who you were before, who you are now and who you will be, and still loving yourself. It is a process that takes a lot of sacrifice and discipline, inside and outside of your life.

It is more than wearing elegant outfits to show off or putting on a smile while chinning up to let people know that you are okay with yourself, when in reality, you are too caught up with how you look, and you hate being seen.

Self-love is the opposite. You appreciate everything within yourself, and more than anything else, you are teaming up with yourself instead of opposing yourself.

Psychologically, loving oneself is such a crucial role in life. It is not at all being narcissistic but being considerate towards others, given the way you live your life in general.

"The beliefs and evaluations people hold about themselves determine who they are, what they can do, and what they can become." (Burns, 1982)

Self-concept is defined as the sum of an individual's beliefs and knowledge about his/her attributes and qualities. It is classified as a cognitive schema that organizes abstract and concrete views about the self and controls the processing of self-relevant information. (Markus, 1977; Kihlstrom and Cantor, 1983)

Therefore, based on the research done by knowledgeable people, together with experiences that the majority of the population go through, self-love is not a mere luxury but a necessity to give significance to in your life.

Chapter 1
The Why of Self-Love

People raising questions, such as those beginning with the "why," would probably lead to others determining that someone is skeptical or doubtful. But in this case, I would like to thank you for thinking that way.

You would *want* to be curious about why self-love is vital and why it has to be a necessity.

Women, as I have experienced all my life as I interact with my relatives and friends of the opposite sex, are more emotional types of people, needing a lot of assurance and affirmation, especially from those closest to them. Although I don't quite grasp all the aspects of womanhood, I do believe there is a big difference between each unique woman in this world.

But then, I also realize that not every woman feels the same about herself. And the very heart of that matter is the subject of this book you're holding right now.

Why do you need self-love if the love and care you get from your family and friends are enough?

Why does self-love feel like something impossible to achieve, especially when you label yourself with all the negative flaws you see in the mirror?

If you think self-love is a selfish act, remember that not loving yourself also means not being able to love others, either.

Right now, I ask you not to shake off your doubts and skepticism, for it may lead you to the light at the end of the tunnel, which is where this book will take you.

Why is Self-Love Essential?

When we were kids, we were constantly asked who's prettier. Our automatic response was, of course, none other than ourselves. It's normal for innocent kids to do so, because, at that early age, their judgment is solely based upon their subjectivity of who comes first— themselves, of course!

Kids are naturally selfish. They want to have the food they like all to themselves. They don't like to have their toys shared with others. The centre of their growing-up years is themselves. That's why they are being taught to give, that "sharing is caring."

But when they've grown up and matured, a lot of other things take up space in their hearts. It includes their family, friends, close relationships, and anything else that would matter to them the most.

As grown-ups, we tend to put ourselves aside and worry about others. We worry when we don't please them because of our limitations and incapacity. We worry when, or if we are not enough for them. We learn to ignore our rights and beliefs, only to put someone else's comfort first. Since we are grown-ups, we ought to be more considerate of everyone else, regardless.

And sometimes we wish we were back to those good old days when we were just being selfish and self-centred. We are tired of giving and bottling up inside what we should've whined about; if only we were back to being a child.

This is why self-love is essential.

It makes us feel like a child again, but only with this differing point of view

: without being selfish.

We miss our childhood days where we were enough for ourselves, and we didn't care about what others would think of us.

We were just fine as we were, and we didn't feel so insisted upon to be like someone else, that we were not.

Because, as reality hits us in the face every day, we are exposed to people-pleasing rather than self-worth building.

As kids, we don't care what people think of us. But today, we give so much importance to other people's opinions about how they perceive us.

We miss being spoiled because now we don't seem to be deserving of anything. We feel like we don't deserve the right to demand, perhaps because we feel like we are not worthy enough. Not yet, anyway.

Given all these fundamental issues, think of how life could get even worse than it is if we don't give importance to loving ourselves.

If you are guilty of these signs, then you need to work on your self-love:

- You readily accept blame, even if it's not your fault.

- You think you don't deserve to be praised for the efforts you have made.

- You don't focus on the good things you have.

- You keep yourself indulged in the negatives.

- You keep losing hope. You also keep pulling yourself down from having high hopes again.

- You loathe everything about yourself, in detail.

- You care for others less than for yourself, thinking you are just worthless.

Obviously, if you are guilty of one or all of the above, you are basically on the opposite side of the fence to where this book is going.

Instead of healthily living with self-love, you live under your self- restraints— thinking you deserve nothing less than that.

Now that I have expressed the profundity of why self-love is essential through the apparent effects of losing it, you may want to ask yourself: Do you still see self-love as nothing but an outward accessory?

As much as it is that too, without self-love, your life will continually be disintegrating in the darkness of your own self-made, unworthy interpretation of yourself.

So instead of asking why self-love is essential, let yourself rather ask, why not?

Why is it so hard to practice?

"Loving yourself truly, comes with facing what you may hate most about yourself. Maybe it is a body part or multiple body parts, or the way you treated someone or guilt or shame about a situation. The thing is, until you can shine a light on your insecurities, you will never be truly accepting of yourself," says Dr. Allison Apfelbaum.

Dr. Apfelbaum laid a firm foundation here about our hatred of certain parts of ourselves, resulting in a lack of self-love, or the total absence of it.

In a sense, you find yourself in a catch-22 situation, where it probably means because of your lack of love for yourself, you keep shaming your body. But also, because of your body shape, you keep losing self-love. That's why you keep body-shaming yourself.

The hatred towards ourselves dominates our ability to appreciate ourselves more because we think if we were more attractive we would be motivated to be better.

The only way to overcome an enemy is to face it--conquering it head-on and making it bow down to our commands.

And your enemy, would not be anything from the outside other than your lying, deceptive brain speaking to you. It may look like an ally, but when it becomes your source of self-loathing instead of self-loving and healthy mental preservation, it becomes your greatest enemy.

You are the only one in control of your brain, and whether it is thinking this way or not, is your responsibility and choice. In other words, your adversary to conquer is yourself, and no other.

You know in your mind that you are the one putting the burden on your shoulders because you think it would lessen the self-loathing. But guess what? It does not. One way or another, it only makes things worse than ever.

It makes you lose your confidence in all other aspects of your life and creeps into your manifestations and daily life.

"We think if we punish ourselves enough, we'll change. Accepting ourselves unconditionally is difficult because we must give up the <u>fantasy</u> that if we punish ourselves enough with negative thoughts, we'll change." -<u>Barbara Markway Ph.D.</u>

This is such a common excuse we use to continually justify our actions. There is this fantasy that we're always seeking change but never really going after it in the right direction, as Dr. Markway deliberated.

Do you see this point? How hard have we been on ourselves when we lack something, commit errors, and overreact to things? But when it comes to others, we become like compassionate nuns who extend such patience just to be considerate to them and their faults.

Now, you've pretty much understood what makes self-love so hard to practice. You're probably thinking of ways to get the better of it and conquer what has been holding you back from really living an extraordinary life, filled with self-love and affirmation.

But let me affirm once again why this book holds special significance for telling women of their value. It is such an obvious topic since women play an amazing role in the economic and social world, and therefore, it is only right to affirm the value of every single woman, who they really are, and what they can do.

Chapter 2
Know Your Vulnerabilities

Before we move to our main point, let us first get a clear view of what it means to know our vulnerabilities.

Say you are up for a battle with your physical enemies like in a mobile game or a group of gangsters, your vulnerabilities would mean, your weak points you have, to protect you during the game. So, before digging into the actual attack, you have to keep it safe from such stimuli that would weaken you into losing.

But here's the catch. Your enemy is yourself, and that enemy knows of your vulnerabilities well enough, more than your conscious mind does. It's too confusing, right? At the sound of it, you probably thought that you might have two personalities inside, which is common and understandable for us humans to assume.

So now, you have to figure out how to protect your weakest points from being attacked by your deceitful mind.

How is that possible, you thought?

Dear reader friend, it's as simple as 1, 2, 3.

You just have to wake up and become aware of it. You know it already because your enemy knows it, and your enemy is you. You just have to accept that those are your weaknesses and become fully awakened to the fact that you cannot change it as it is, but you can control how you protect it and react when things have gone out of control concerning your weaknesses.

Don't be too blinded by other people's standard-setting for you or the type of "someone" you want to become that's too far removed from who you are.

Humans are created to be uniquely and amazingly different from each other. Here's how it works in a smaller picture. Dogs don't compare themselves with cats. They don't meow like cats, and cats don't bark like something they're not. They are simply living the way they are created to be. And that's how it is with us also.

Our minds, which become our enemies, bring us so many doubts and terrible suggestions because we think that it may at least help us become someone better than we are. That's toxicity.

That is why we have to become aware of our vulnerabilities so that finally, we can start addressing ourselves from the heart of the matter.

How do you get to know your specific weaknesses? Of course, you can never find the answers to other people's opinions. You know, therefore, try asking the right questions of yourself.

1. When do I get offended the most?

2. What are the things I hate and the things that make me sad?

3. Who are the people that help worsen my mental and emotional health?

4. What are the habits and negative thoughts that keep ruining me?

5. Who am I?

These are guiding questions you can begin with, to know more about yourself and your vulnerabilities. However, it doesn't stop there. You might want to get to know more about yourself every single day, by spending an ample amount of time evaluating your thoughts.

Similarly, I'm sure you have your brain muscles working by now. But remember not to get too uptight! There are no wrong answers. . You just have to ask the correct, more positive questions.

Have you been well lately? What are the things that keep triggering you?

Questions that are smooth and kind are ones you also deserve to ask. Now begin with yourself.

Accept your weakness

There are many tips and suggestions people threw at us when we were growing up, especially at most counselling sessions (and some that we didn't even ask for.) But what was there to help us accept our weaknesses when we ought to have been strong and not dumbstruck by our vulnerability, every single time?

1. Accepting your weaknesses means recognizing that you are not your flaws. That's all there is to it. You are not the time when you cried so much

because you didn't understand what was in the lesson in your music class. You know better than that. It was just a part of you, not all of you.

2. Accept your weakness and don't cover it up with shame, self-hate, and regret. That makes it very, very uncool. Instead, start showing it and working out its every angle for improvement. Say, "this is my weakness and I am not ashamed of it; it's a part of me and I don't have to be sorry that it is." Then, while you keep embracing it like that, you will eventually start loving how you feel about yourself if you just keep being honest.

3. Your weaknesses are not your endpoint. As a matter of fact, your weakness now, wouldn't have to matter ten years from today. And on top of that, it could even become your

greatest strength! That happened to me, and strictly speaking, it is never impossible. Here's why. Just imagine you have an obvious lack of talent, like not knowing how to cook well, and your food tastes awful. Because of that, you are stressing about when you will ever be able to taste the delicious food you cooked. And then, unconsciously, you keep doing and trying your best to make your food taste a little better than the tasteless meals before. Until it just happened, after many years of stressing over unpalatable meals you have mastered and excelled at cooking. That's just such a wow moment! A story like that can happen to anyone who struggles with their weaknesses. You see, your strengths are already honed. They are already strengths that might need a little brushing up. But it doesn't mean you should neglect it already. You should not only focus on the gaps, but also on the bridges that can close the gaps to your abilities.

How to overcome toxic emotions

Toxic emotions:

"A general term for negative emotions, such as stress and anger, which harm a person's mental and, possibly, physical health."

Emotions are neither good nor bad. Not even neutral. They are the results of our subjective minds and are, therefore, not rational. However, when our emotions come to the point where it leads to our downfall, ineffectiveness, and unproductivity, that's when it becomes toxic.

Emotions don't have the final word on us. We should have a grasp on our feelings instead. As I said, they are not neutral;

they are controllable and able to be disciplined, and it is up to us and our choices, how we are going to manage such overwhelmingly strong feelings.

Anger, frustration, resentment, and all the other negative emotions may take their toll on us and make us eventually break down. You might think how this significantly affects us in loving ourselves, right?

When we feel too much, stress out heavily, or are on the verge of an emotional breakdown, we become very irrational. We barely understand anything about ourselves. And this results in hating ourselves instead of raising our morale at that point. Emotions can be very deceptive.

It even creeps into the stability that we worked so hard to achieve. Even the pattern and stable ground we consistently worked so hard on, loving ourselves and taking care of ourselves, are in danger when our bottled-up, toxic emotions bursts forth and we only have a thread to hold onto.

These toxic emotions, wherever they are sourced from, if it happens to be entertained and not appropriately managed, tend to be very destructive to our self-esteem, confidence and even the very thing that helps pull ourselves together. At the end of the day, we just find ourselves back at the beginning again, broken into pieces and wrecked, as if a fiery storm has passed by.

Knowing its root is the very thing you have to illuminate in your mind first, before really conquering it. And yes, you have all the right and power to overcome it, even if you think it's already overcoming you. You are the navigator of your mind, so learn to control its cunning and devious tactics.

Overcoming these overwhelming feelings that eat away at us, is not simply managing how to get out of it or "unfeeling it." It may take a while, but trust the process of learning how to recognize that you are *feeling* these emotions, "determining *why* we are feeling this way, and allowing ourselves to *receive the messages* that they are sending us before we release them and move forward. Yes, that statement may sound a little odd, but our emotions are designed to be messengers to tell us something. These messages can be very valuable if we listen."

—Elizabeth Scott, MS

As complicated as these emotions might be, you have to have a very strong drive not to let them reign. Use some time to feel something else by being productive. Spending time with friends can also distract you from such all-consuming thoughts that are so heavy to carry.

Especially to most women, to whom emotional issues are much more prominent, given that they are the kind who feel much more complicated emotions than guys do.

After all, overcoming negativities and toxic emotions all depend on your choices and determination. You choose whether to react to it or not or to react positively and productively, or not. You choose whether to convert all the forces of these toxic emotions into something valuable and fruitful, such as working out, heavy exercises or even writing. You can always be creative in ways that consume your energy.

That is one good way of overcoming it. You're not forcing it to be driven away with all your might, but instead, you are turning it into something more innovative. As I said, these toxic emotions, when handled wisely, in the right way, can produce a result that can even boost your self-love. It's recycling the emotions that might harm you and turning them into things that would be beneficial to your physical and mental health.

You are then benefitting twice when you choose to handle your rage or strong toxic emotions properly. Or should I say "killing two birds with one stone?"

Firstly, you are eliminating the toxicity in your mind and feelings. And secondly, but not least, you are making the most of it instead of getting wrecked by it. It all depends on how you face it and handle it. It's just a matter of decisions—letting rationality win over emotions that are not constructive enough to be entertained.

How is it worth it

Now that you've reached almost the end of chapter two, some thoughts might be uppermost in your mind.

Why is everything, from what we've discussed above, worth doing and applying? Well, I guess that's why you picked up this book—because you got interested when you read the word "self-love," knowing that that's the very thing you lack.

Let me pat you on the back. That's correct! And should I take this space and time to remind you that you should remember, all along, why you picked up this book and continued reading until now because you want to love yourself? After all, who wouldn't? And when everybody else does this and that, and hates and loves, who would want to love you first, if not you, right?

Before you find yourself being loved by anybody from outside, learn to love yourself first because everything will follow on perfectly when you do.

Let me tell you that the moment you have learned and stabilized the foundations of loving yourself, you will never allow anybody to define how you should be treated, for you know in yourself that you are to be loved and respected and, with due respect, acknowledged. You would never need to seek love in the wrong places again, for you have enough love for yourself. You have the regard and care that you deserve and people around you would appreciate how much self-esteem you radiate with your presence. Self-love impacts a woman's life much more than anything that can be given to her. Can you imagine how much that is worth pondering? About becoming a woman who has unlocked the power which makes

her beautiful and productive in her unique
way?

Chapter 3
Road to Self-Love

Should I guess how you got here? You have desired so much in your heart to love yourself, right?

If I got that spot on, then you should keep diving deeper into this book. And congratulate yourself for reaching the mid-point on this subject here.

Now that we have discussed our vulnerabilities, how to accept our flaws and weaknesses, and how to win over our toxic emotions, we should finally get to the lighter aspects of our discussion.

I am sure you're with me on this one— that love is the most significant and purest act we can offer anyone. It's powerful to the point that it can drive every aspect of us—

mentally, physically, spiritually, and emotionally.

Now, let me ask you a favour. I want you to picture this in your mind as vividly as you can. Think about how much you love someone, romantically. Focus your thoughts on that person at the other end, receiving your love. Tell him how much you love him and how much you care. And do we love with words alone? We prove it through actions and everything that pleases the subject of our love. You only do things that make him happy.

Now, stop the daydreaming, and let's get back to reality concerning self-love.

Do you love yourself the way you love the person in your imagination? Or the person you're in a relationship with?

Expose yourself to colours.

I should compliment you with how creative your imagination was about picturing someone you love. Even if it's only in your mind, I'm sure you would feel butterflies and great desire in your heart. It's good and, no doubt, healthy.

The very reason why you should also love yourself, to the extent you can love others, is for exactly that reason.

Because it's not just healthy, it heals every part of you and calms everything that once enraged you about yourself. Once, you indulged yourself with self-loathing, now you have illuminated yourself with colours that would shine the brightest around you.

Can you even imagine a world without colours? That's how we were when we didn't know about loving ourselves. We lived in darkness, walking by mere chance and almost stumbling every time and everywhere. We never liked colourless things. It's too dull. Too boring.

Here's why that's important. You start painting yourself with colours that beam wonderful glowing hues to others, resulting in them being attracted to you, like an elegant sunflower in a field of flowers.

That's how self-love works. And it suits you magnificently. It's a beautiful ornament that is not just a luxury, but always a necessity to wear.

When you wear self-love and become so attached to it that it's finally found to be engraved in your heart, your sparkle would be constant, even in your darkest night. Just as you don't easily give up on someone you love, you also wouldn't know giving up as a choice for yourself. You have been trained to be strong because self-love will be in the blood that flows through your veins

That doesn't mean it will cure you of all the bad days ahead of you. Self-love doesn't mean you're not going to commit any more mistakes than before, and you will always be kind to yourself. Nor does it mean such instant healing and immunity from bitterness. It won't eliminate your weaknesses.

It just means you will always choose the better option, if not the best for yourself. You choose what suits you perfectly. You choose the rainbow when all is dark around you. You choose to open up to trustworthy friends and trust them to be with you through the process, instead of locking yourself away in isolation. You choose to care for yourself even when no one else does or when you don't feel like it. You choose to compliment yourself, even when you feel like there's nothing to be complimented about.

You just want to indulge yourself with colours instead of the darkness this world brings you. Because you know there will come a time that problems and hardships will end, and you are looking forward to that. Such colours are preparations that you are positive enough to make for all the good things you deserve, even after going through storms and sinking boats.

Self-love is what makes you stand out— because you started to be you, to wear the colours that define who you are, to stop the pretense and start showing off your natural face, unhidden by the mask.

Self-love begins in knowing your true colours and being proud of them. It's not narcissistic, since you acknowledge all the gaps there are for your improvement. You just acknowledge that your mistakes and flaws and your imperfections are fitting together all the pieces of who you are meant to be, marvellously.

They are there to complement your true colours. Once you get used to self-love, your light will illuminate these naturally, because you finally love the colours of your likeness—the colours you expose yourself to, the colours that reflect you best.

Celebrate yourself

Another significant way of manifesting how wonderfully you love yourself is by celebrating who you have been, who you are now, and who you will be shortly. Because you now believe that abandoning yourself will only lead to a scary place, like depression and hopelessness. You choose to just be you. Improve who you are. Work out yourself for the betterment of your own life. And you will stop copying who others are since the comparison is such a poisonous act that would creep you out and cripple your beliefs about yourself.

You are celebrating yourself because you are made to be unique, and no one else is made to be like you, not even your mother or your sibling.

There are tiny, but grand ways to celebrate yourself and your existence every day:

1. Appreciate that it is only grace that makes you breathe and your heartbeat every second. Therefore, learn to thank the Lord for your life and all your resources and abilities that keep you going.
2. Treat yourself with regard, exceptional care, and any healthy food you crave. Yes, treat yourself when you feel down or when you feel happy. Learn to be content spending time in your own company. You are your own best friend and helper, after all.
3. Spend time with those who make you happy, the people who inspire you,

and love you the way you should be loved. Join your friends for a girls' night out. Strengthen your relationships and solidify your connections. They are blessings that bring additional wonders to your life.

4. Write a list of what makes you happy and do it. Pick some flowers. Read a book or watch that Netflix series that stirred your interest. Go enjoy the sun and the calm of the beach. Satisfy yourself to your heart's content. You deserve it, after all, for surviving this far in your life.

5. Enhance your passion and keep doing it. I promise, whatever it is—whether it be beauty, music, writing, sports, or any recreational or health inclined activities—make it your hobby and share it with the world. That's where you shine and that's incredible!

Chapter 4
A Lifetime Journey

Just as the way you love someone, your family, a friend, or a lifetime partner, that is how you also need to love yourself. You don't decide to start loving yourself at one point and end at another. It keeps going on and on, as long as you have breath and life and everything that keeps you going as you.

Self-love is not a one-time decision. It never will be. You have to keep choosing it, every time. You have to keep siding with loving yourself, making it a constant in your life. Or else you will find yourself losing the game again.

Once you learn to win the battle of choosing self-love every day, it's time for you to burn the bridges. Never go back to the old habits of who you were. Keep choosing to grow in it, to grow the love you have for yourself, and you will reap the harvest of how well-cared for and nourished you have been. Because the little steps of choosing self-love brought you to the place of no-return, you will reap the pedestal, where you will have the privilege to be the centre of your life.

You are not meant to be an empty cup.

How many times a day do we have to sacrifice ourselves for another, say a responsibility or a person? And at sunset, when the long day is finally over, you will find yourself emptied and exhausted. The week has passed by, and you remain the same empty cup you were, while people going in and out of your life keep demanding and asking you for more.

That's how we busy-bees are. We keep sacrificing and doing more, even to the full extent of ourselves. We even forget how to refill the energy that's been lost. Just how am I going to be whole again, we ask?

But, have you ever asked yourself, why are you doing that? Why do you keep emptying your cup, only to fill others' cups?

In a world where beating ourselves up and productivity is normal and acceptable, how many times did people ever greet us happily when we cancelled great plans that we knew would eventually drain us? Did we ever get to hear someone congratulate us when we chose to sleep and rest, over accepting that ample opportunity knocking on our door, that requires more energy than we can give?

That's weird, right? No one would. We never did.

We tend to just dive into the deepest ocean and just not worry about how we are going to breathe once we've used up all our oxygen. We just have to beat ourselves up a little more than before. "Maybe I can do it." And sooner, while we're at it, we'll ask. "How did it get this bad?"

Well, we always choose things that will eventually lead to burnout because "that's how I am going to be more productive."

Does it lead to healthy productivity, when you insist on pouring from an empty cup?

There are fruitful ways to be productive, without exhausting yourself. It just comes with the proper perspective. When you start standing on this principle that you are not meant to be an empty cup, shallow, deserted, and unattended, you'll somehow start valuing self-love over compromising.

Choose yourself first

Here's how the Direction Psychology Social Worker, Joseph Fleming, put it:

"Self-care is the conscious effort of making time for activities you find beneficial in maintaining your mental and physical health. Caring for your mind and body doesn't have to be time-consuming but does require regular and ongoing attention. Eating and drinking well, getting enough sleep, exercising, avoiding alcohol and drugs, and living a healthy, active lifestyle are just some of the physical health-related aspects of self-care. But don't forget to focus on the mental health aspects too, like relaxation, mindfulness, social connections, and hobbies.

Your health is invaluable, and your self-care can't afford to wait. If you keep putting others first, you'll soon find that you don't have anything left to give them. Sometimes looking after yourself is the best gift you can give to others."

To other people, choosing yourself first would mean acting very selfishly.

But that's not how it works. There are just some people who don't know the concept of loving oneself. When you are choosing yourself first, you are saying that you value who you are and that you don't need to give a damn about anything that causes you to stress out.

You are just protecting the thing that keeps your mental health and emotional state in balance. Never permit anyone to judge you as being "selfish" just because you are prioritizing your wellness first.

Again, let me raise this question: Is it even okay to drain yourself for someone else's good and happiness but not protect yourself from being exhausted, peaceless, or unstable?

What I mean by this is that you are freeing yourself from anything that would make you feel like a captive in bondage. You are always choosing what's better for you so you can also do better, and even great things for others because you chose to take care of your issues and stability first. You're fully present in yourself, and when that happens, you'll simply overflow and give people around you the joy and peace you have within.

Know your worth and radiate it

More than anything else in this world, knowing your worth is the most important thing that keeps you from neglecting who you are. You don't let anybody else invalidate you, your feelings, your esteem, your personality, or anything.

You already have the firm ground of knowing that you're worth more than any material possessions you own. Your value cannot be measured by money or anything the world can offer, and you know you'll never settle for anything less, anymore.

Because you know your worth, you try to always be the best version of yourself, expecting that those good things will only follow later. You've set your standards for the best, and always noble and excellent things are your goals.

You surely know that you know yourself better than anyone else, and no one could ever be compared to you. That's why you don't look for another to give you the definition of who you are because you are enough.

When you've already worked on loving yourself, you will find out that not everyone deserves your attention. Not everyone deserves to be in your life. You have been okay with simply cutting people out to protect your heart.

You've learned to be fine with your own company, even without the presence of somebody else. You are your biggest fan. You're okay, even when people don't like you because you started to like yourself first.

Since you are in control of your happiness, you'll never get lonely anymore when on your own. You choose yourself since you know what you deserve, and you won't settle for anything that could only cause you chaos.

Since you know your value already, you will only keep attracting the best things. You'll radiate and overflow with the grace that people will just naturally see in you. It's easier to give because your heart is settled, and your hands are full of love and care for yourself. You acknowledge that whoever comes for you, is for you, and whoever leaves is eventually the one who never gets to see your worth. You're okay with anything, as long as it's for the best for you.

Chapter 5
Meet the Stronger You

Hey! What's up? How have you been doing? Oh, nice biceps there. Your core looks good. What a nice body! You must've worked out hard, huh?

Yes, that's it. That's what people say whenever they see someone with an attractive, healthy body, such as a gym enthusiast. You've got some muscles to flex, of course! And wouldn't you be proud of that? That's just the result of hard work, discipline, and uh ... you know what else when you've been working out!

The goal? The goal is to look good and strengthening your physique!

Well, dear female reader, that's just the same as you do when you practice self-love. You not only look good, but you also manifest strength and power. And, oh, the hard work you put in for yourself all along.

Of course, the only difference is that you just don't do it for other people now. You do it for yourself, for you to meet the more robust you, the stable and maturing you.

Similar to going to the gym, you had to "work out" as well. Hard work, perseverance, consistency, and the determination of the will to just continue on because you are sure that somehow, someday, soon, you are going to meet the stronger you. Someone who doesn't know the words "giving up."

No, it does not mean the stronger you are, the fewer your weaknesses will be. You'll probably be aware of having times when you still stumble and lose your balance, and that is fine. Even birds lose sight and balance. But now, you are more capable of helping yourself up, not needing a hand or anybody's assistance any longer. You've acquired strength and power that you would never find from somebody else. You've raised your expectations and standards when it comes to people, and first and foremost, you trust yourself. In loving yourself you have a long way to go, but you are in the centre now, come what may, where there's consistency.

It's okay to be yourself.

On the way to loving yourself, the only key is consistency. Your worth and value are absolute; your colours won't change because that's who you are, and the only controllable thing you can manage is how you feel about, and see yourself. You might have gone through despair and self-loathing before you picked up this book, and dear reader, I won't reprimand you for that. It only means you have a lot more to know about yourself such that would amaze you to the extent that would definitely change your view of yourself.

Now, I want you to imagine again loving somebody else, a person you are in love with, maybe.

That person feels insecure about their appearance, their voice, their hair, and everything else about themselves, and yet, you don't care. You still choose to love them despite the insecurities that they define themselves as. You focus on who they are and not their flaws. You love them with all your heart because, despite everything, you still do. Right? Is that how you feel?

It's such a fantastic kind of love, isn't it? A love that is not based upon the performance of the other but upon your decision to do so because you simply love the person.

Dear woman, I hope that goes for you too. I hope you don't focus on what you define yourself to be but on who you are. I hope you truly realize that it is okay to be yourself. You are an amazing person. I believe people around you see it already, so don't be blinded by your prejudice toward yourself.

Be that first person who's your biggest fan. Be the person who loves you above anything else and despite everything. Be someone who pats you on the back when you fail and treats you to fancy dinners when you win or when success steps in. Be the person who thinks you deserve flowers, extra care, and healthy love, like how parents love their children. Be the person who looks after you, and makes your coffee, lets you rest after a long heavy day, and affirms you with such calming, assuring words. Be that first person to love yourself. Don't wait for anybody else to do it for you.

Besides, if you can do that for another person, why can't you do it for yourself?

Trust yourself. Trust the process.

And even more, look for inspirations from people who have gone a long way in loving themselves first. See how they have blossomed in self-love and how it affected others around them. Believe that it is also yours to claim and practice because self-love is such a wonderful personal power. It is in there, waiting to be awakened.

It's okay to be different from all the others.

It's okay if you belong to the minority of people who choose silence over Friday partying. It's okay if you don't have a partner right now because you choose maturity and self-love first over heartbreak. It's okay if you don't get along well with people you meet for the first time, or if you have distinct eating habits. Whoever you are, even if you don't belong to the majority of people, it doesn't make you the least of these.

You are unique, with every strand of hair on your head and every word you speak.

No one could be matched to your DNA. No one could picture your favourite book more than you. No one could play such harmonious music more than you can.

So who you are, whatever race or family you come from, no one can take away the approval you deserve to have. The only approval and esteem that matters are from yourself. As long as you have you, it's all worth it.

You might be wondering how to stay on track in this journey you started for yourself. These are thoughts you have to tell yourself--simple ways to remind you that you are valuable and that you don't need to lose it. So, encourage yourself. Tell yourself sweet things you want to hear from others. Your voice matters, too.

1. "I love you, and I'm happy to be you."

These are the words you should always tell yourself. And live it out. Love yourself in action. Start with simple ones, like caring for your hair and your skin, to delving into deep routines, like resting and healthy soul meditations.

2. "I'm proud of how far you've come."

It may be your work journey or the skills you're trying to progress in, or just holding onto life; look back and trace the little steps you took and see the miles and miles you've walked, just to be here where you are now. It's an enormous reason to boast.

3. "You know, Self, I trust in you. It's okay to make mistakes. I'm always here to accept and forgive you."

By saying this, you are acknowledging that mistakes and failures are inevitable along the way, and you don't cut off the possibilities that you're going to stumble. But you don't always expect to stumble. In contrast, you are gentle with yourself by saying that whatever happens, it's okay.

It's still worth it. You're still valuable, even if you're still a work in progress. You clearly assure yourself that you can always extend forgiveness to yourself for what you've done wrong. It's okay to blame yourself but for just a little while, and then carry on trying again.

4. "I'm going to be mindful of my limitations while challenging myself to new adventures."

This is a healthy way of resting and gliding through life. You know your limits, and you are going to venture into new paths, skills, or grow in something you've never tried before. By doing this, you are giving yourself the liberty to enjoy the rest of what's out in the world by not neglecting and sacrificing your boundaries.

Specially you

What are your dreams for yourself?

Ten years from today, what kind of clothes would you be wearing? A medical robe? Maternity clothes? You might think that you're too late to dream up something new again. But is it? Do you dream of owning a café or a garden bookstore? Do you dream of getting married in Italy or somewhere in New York?

Why would your dreams be invalidated?

It is you--in particular, after all...

No one has the same dream as you do. No one can love as you love. No one has the same reason or purpose as you because you are complex but profound, and yet so simple but elegant. You are a paradox no one can understand, but also an open book.

No one's story could inspire other people like your story does. And no one has the same "memory lane" like yours.

Since you are an individual with intrinsic worth, it gives you the key to unlock your identity to being a woman of power, equipped with self-love.

No chances, opportunities, open doors can come to another the same as it comes to you. Variables, such as people around you are, as a matter of fact, hardly ever the same as another. In this world, you barely would meet anyone who walks, eats, dances, sings, and cares as you do, and you'll only exhaust yourself trying to find one. Not even twins can be precisely the same.

My point here is, you are who you are specially made to be. No one can grab your purpose and meaning and wear it on themselves, nor can you do it for other people. The only thing you can powerfully do for yourself is live it. Living it is loving it. You'll find yourself loving the way you are, the way you breathe life in this world.

Apologies, but shouldn't you start loving yourself now? In an honest manner?

Conclusion

Hey! Let's shake hands on coming this far in your desire to nurture this new journey. I say you're doing yourself a favour, big time, for picking this book up and reading it till the end. I am confident that you are already feeling a burning sensation in your heart, saying to yourself that once you put down this book, you'll start living in a new world. You'll replace your lenses with the perspective of self-love. You'll start manifesting it and showing the world how you radiate your intrinsic worth and individuality, beginning in your simple ways.

Before this exposition ends, I want to remind you of all the knowledge and memories you picked up while walking throughout the pages of this book. Plant it in your mind and let it grow. Take it everywhere you go and speak it out loud. Share the love you have within you and the power that's begging to be awakened. And as you awaken it, do not be dismayed because you are now becoming the woman of power, of capacity, and grace that you want to be.

And keep these things in mind:

1. You have the inner power within you that only you can discover and awaken.

2. Learning to love yourself may be a long journey, but remember that you're always nearing the goal. Get out and read the map. You're getting there, finally.

3. Catch up with people who also love themselves in different and unique ways. Be influenced by their positivity.

4. Know your colours, stick with them and radiate them. You are a spectrum of colours, and you have to shine your hue.

5. Create your unique style. You know best what defines you, and whatever it is, it is beautiful.

6. Affirm yourself in your mind and out loud. Look in the mirror and encourage yourself to be someone who you want to be today. You'll eventually become someone special whom you'll manifest.

7. Speak out loud when you share your progress with others. Listen to how you are proud of your small steps, and whatever their reactions are, know that the only opinion that matters is yours. Yet still, you learned to accept compliments.

8. Learn the techniques of what therapy will work best for you. Run to it when you begin to have those dark clouds and do not give in. Instead, fight.

9. Celebrate yourself, not just on bright days, but every single day.

10. Learn to cut out people that drain your energy. Know your worth and never settle for anything less.

11. Live easily, putting sobriety before emotions and wisdom before irrationality and prejudice.

12. Choose people who choose you. Know when to open and close doors to anyone, whoever they might be.

13. Above all, protect your heart and then you'll be happy with yourself, having all the love you deserve.

Now, as we end this venture of self-love, I want you to go back to the first line you read in the content of this book. The introductory line. Did you see it? What did you think when you first read it, versus now that you read the total thoughts of the book? Did it summarize everything you read about here?

"Love yourself and everything falls into line."

How glorious that would be, to see it happen in reality! Imagine your life becoming organized and settled because you took that courage to walk that narrow bridge of self-love. Now commit to yourself that there's no turning back, and burn that bridge.

Start manifesting that power within you, dear woman, and see what wonders it will do if you will only begin to live the life of loving yourself. Not only a few things will fall into line, but everything.

Contentment, wisdom, people, and peace, you name it! Self-love cures and heals; who'd have thought that it could also prevent?

Just dive in and see for yourself!

But wait, here's a challenge for you: Why don't you start discovering your ways and means of loving yourself? Self-experiments have become more effective than those imposed on us. Furthermore, you know what kind of person you are, so you'll easily spot where, and what type of coping mechanisms you need. I hope you enjoy trying out things for yourself and knowing how to love yourself, for who you are, fully!

Bibliography

Apfelbaum, Dr. Allison. Why is self-love so difficult?

https://www.kirklandreporter.com/life/why-is-self-love-is-sodifficult/#:~:text=Loving%20yourself%20truly%20comes%20with,be%20truly%20accepting%20of%20yourself.

Scott, Elizabeth,MS.   How Negative Emotions Affect Us.

https://www.verywellmind.com/embrace-negative-emotions-4158317

Fleming, Joseph.   Direction Psychology Social Worker.

You can't pour from an empty cup.
https://www.directionpsychology.com/article/you-cant-pour-from-an-empty-cup/

Kooser, Allison. *Empowered Women Change*

The World. *https://opportunity.org/news/blog/201 7/03/empowered-women-change-the-world*

Markway, Barbara, Ph.D. *Why is self-acceptance so hard.* https://www.psychologytoday.com/us/bl og/shyness-is-nice/201109/why-is-self-acceptance-so-hard

Michal (Michelle) Mann, Clemens M. H. Hosman, Herman P. Schaalma, Nanne K. de Vries. Self-esteem in a broad-spectrum approach for mental health promotion Health Education Research, Volume 19, Issue 4, August 2004, Pages 357–372,

https://doi.org/10.1093/her/cyg041

Rebecca. *Choosing yourself: 10 reasons why it's important*

https://www.minimalismmadesimple.co
m/home/choosing-yourself/

Segen's Medical Dictionary. © 2012 Farle
x, Inc. All rights reserved.
https://medical-
dictionary.thefreedictionary.com/toxic+e
motion#:~:text=A%20general%20term%
20for%20negative,mental%20and%20po
ssibly%20physical%20health

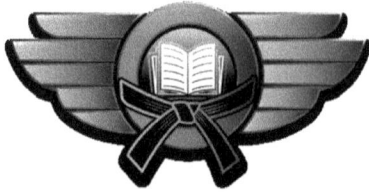

Thank you for reading this book!

If you found this book helpful, I would be grateful if you would **post an honest review on Amazon** so this book can reach other supportive readers like you!

All you need to do is digitally flip to the back and leave your review. Or visit amazon.com/author/senseipauldavid click the correct book cover and click on the blue link next to the yellow stars that says, "customer reviews."

As always...

It's a great day to be alive!

Get/Share Our FREE All-Ages Mental Health Books Now!

FREE Kids Books

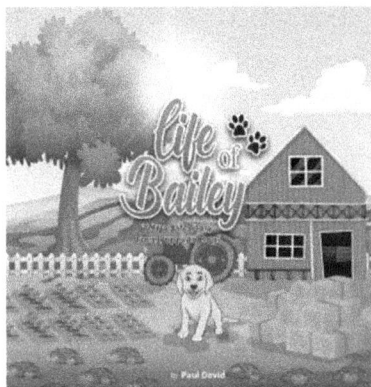

lifeofbailey.senseipublishing.com   kidsonearth.senseipublishing.com

FREE Self-Development Book for Every Family

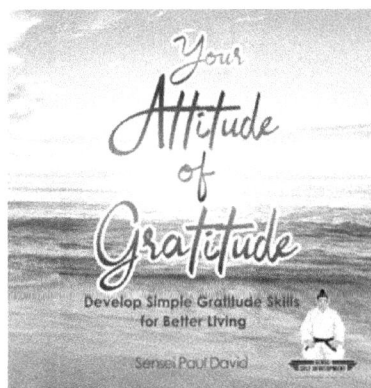

senseiselfdevelopment.senseipublishing.com

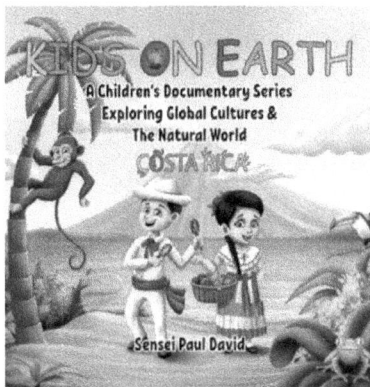

Click Below or Search Amazon for Another Book In Each Series Or Visit:

www.amazon.com/author/senseipauldavid

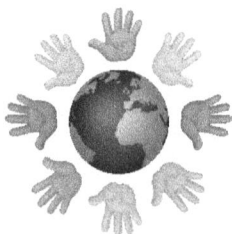

KIDS ON EARTH

kidsonearth.senseipublishing.com

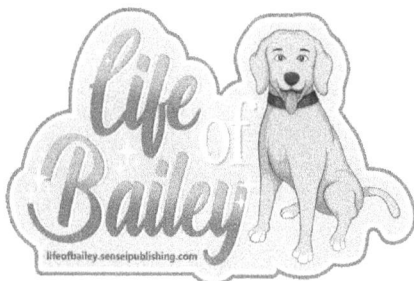

life of Bailey

lifeofbailey.senseipublishing.com

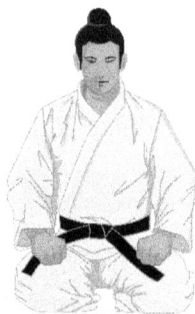

SENSEI SELF DEVELOPMENT
BOOKS SERIES

senseiselfdevelopment.senseipublishing.com

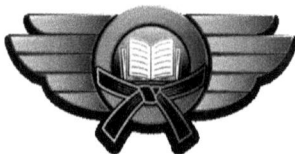

SENSEI PUBLISHING

It's A Great Day To Be Alive!

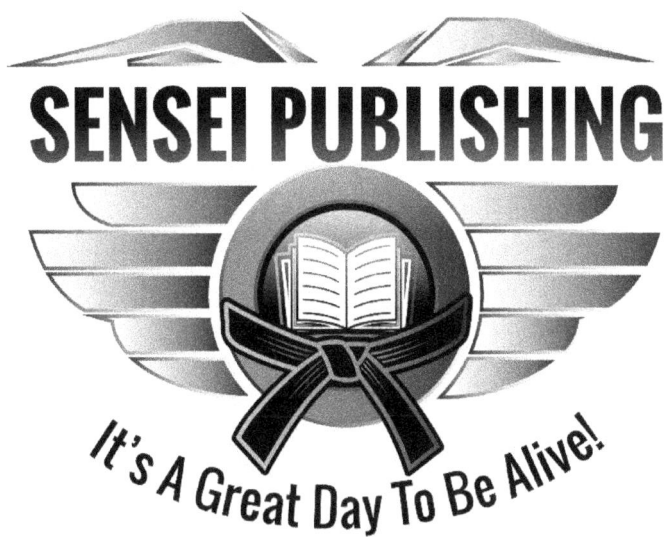

www.senseipublishing.com

@senseipublishing
#senseipublishing

Check out our **recommendations** for
other books for adults & kids plus other
great resources by visiting
www.senseipublishing.com/resources/

Join Our Publishing Journey!

If you would like to receive FREE BOOKS, special offers, please visit www.senseipublishing.com and join our newsletter by entering your email address in the pop-up box

Follow Our Engaging Blog NOW! senseipauldavid.ca

Get Our FREE Books Today!

Click & Share the Links Below

FREE Kids Books

lifeofbailey.senseipublishing.com
kidsonearth.senseipublishing.com

FREE Self-Development Book

senseiselfdevelopment.senseipublishing.com

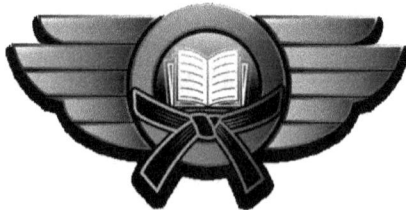

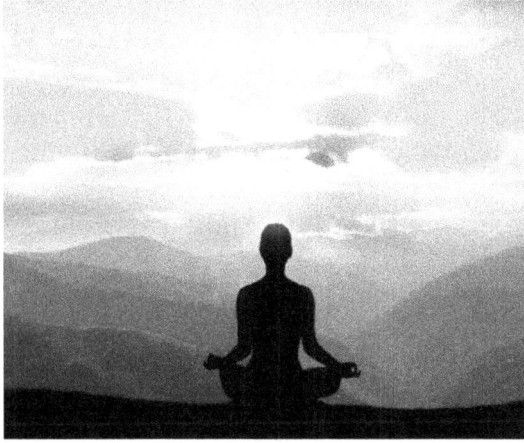

FREE BONUS!!!
Experience Over 25 FREE Engaging Guided Meditations!

Prized Skills & Practices for Adults & Kids. Help Restore Deep-Sleep, Lower Stress, Improve Posture, Navigate Uncertainty & More.

Download the Free Insight Timer App and click the link below:
http://insig.ht/sensei_paul

If you like these meditations & want to go deeper email me for a FREE 30min LIVE Coaching Session:
senseipauldavid@senseipublishing.com

About Sensei Publishing

Sensei Publishing commits itself to help people of all ages transform into better versions of themselves by providing high-quality and research-based self-development books with an emphasis on mental health and guided meditations. Sensei Publishing offers well-written e-books, audiobooks, paperbacks and online courses that simplify complicated but practical topics in line with its mission to inspire people towards positive transformation.

It's a great day to be alive!

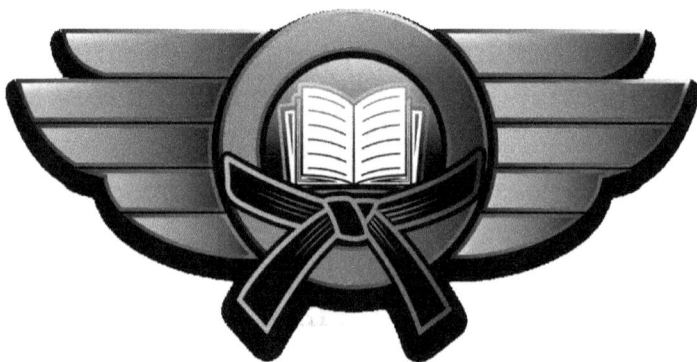

About the Author

I create simple & transformative eBooks & Guided Meditations for Adults & Children proven to help navigate uncertainty, solve niche problems & bring families closer together.

I'm a former finance project manager, private pilot, jiu-jitsu instructor, musician & former University of Toronto Fitness Trainer. I prefer a science-based approach to focus on these & other areas in my life to stay humble & hungry to evolve. I hope you enjoy my work and I'd love to hear your feedback.

- It's a great day to be alive!
Sensei Paul David

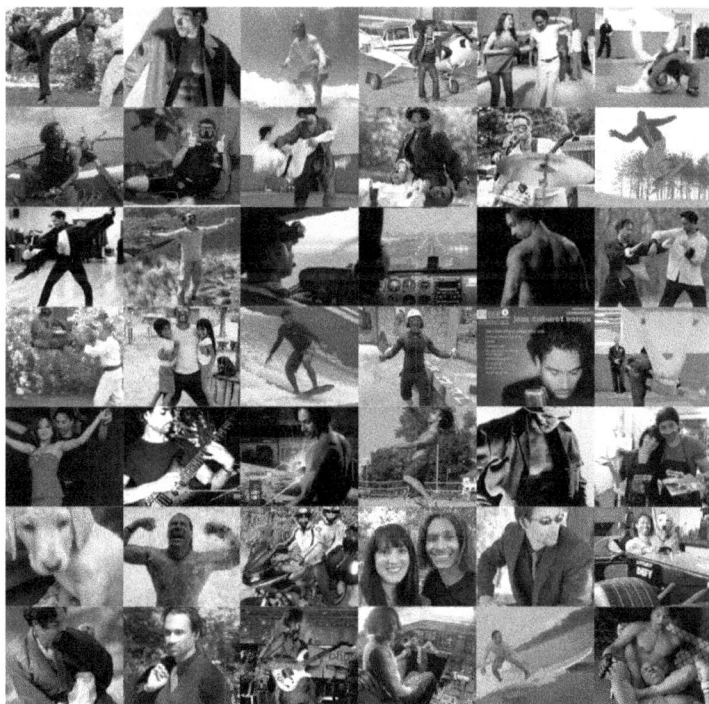

Scan & Follow/Like/Subscribe:
Facebook, Instagram, YouTube:
@senseipublishing

Scan using your phone/iPad camera for Social
Media
Visit us at www.senseipublishing.com and sign
up to our newsletter to learn more about our
exciting books and to experience our FREE
Guided Meditations for Kids & Adults.

www.ingramcontent.com/pod-product-compliance
Lightning Source LLC
Chambersburg PA
CBHW071243020426
42333CB00015B/1605